How To Concentrate Like Einstein:
The Lazy Student's Way to Instantly Improve Memory & Grades with the Doctor Vittoz Secret Concentration Technique.
By Remy Roulier

Copyright © 2012, Remy Roulier

ALL RIGHTS RESERVED. This book contains material protected under International and Federal Copyright Laws and Treaties. Any unauthorized reprint or use of this material is prohibited. No part of this book may be reproduced or transmitted in any form or by any means, electronic or mechanical, including photocopying, recording, or by any information storage and retrieval system without express written permission from the author.

Disclaimer

The author and publisher of this eBook and the associated materials have used their best efforts in preparing this material. The author and publisher make no representations or warranties with respect to the accuracy, applicability, fitness, or completeness of the contents of this material. They disclaim any warranties expressed or implied, merchantability, or fitness for any particular purpose. The author and publisher shall in no event be held liable for any loss or other damages, including but not limited to special, incidental, consequential, or other damages. If you have any doubts about anything, the advice of a competent professional should be sought.

TABLE OF CONTENTS

WELCOME ON BOARD! 5

HOW TO USE THIS BOOK 8

Part 1- A NEW BEGINNING IN LIFE WITH EINSTEIN'S SECRET 9

   a- Concentration: the Key to Success 9

   b- Examples of Successful People with Incredible Focus Ability 14

   c- The Lazy Student's Golden Concentration Formula 16

Part 2- EXPERTS BEST PRACTICES TO IMPROVE THE LAZY STUDENT'S CONCENTRATION 17

   Best Practice 1: HOW TO INSTANTLY RECOVER YOUR POWER OF CONCENTRATION WHEN YOU FEEL STRESSED OR ANXIOUS 17

   Best Practice 2: HOW TO CONCENTRATE TO REDUCE YOUR STUDY TIME BY 3 OR MORE AND INSTANTLY INCREASE YOUR EFFICIENCY 25

   Best Practice 3: HOW YOUR STUDY PLACE CAN INCREASE YOUR CONCENTRATION BY 27% AND MORE IN TWO SIMPLE STEPS 34

   Best Practice 4: HOW TO AVOID GETTING DISTRACTED BY PEOPLE, TV AND OTHER SPARE-TIME ACTIVITIES AND REMAIN FOCUSED 40

   Best Practice 5: HOW TO INSTANTLY STOP YOUR MIND FROM WANDERING WHEN YOU NEED TO CONCENTRATE 42

   Best Practice 6: HOW TO KEEP A FULL CONCENTRATION DURING A THREE HOURS LECTURE 45

Part 3- THE DOCTOR VITTOZ SECRET CONCENTRATION TECHNIQUE 49

   ONE LAST WORD 63

   ABOUT THE AUTHOR 64

MORE BOOKS FROM THE AUTHOR 65

WELCOME ON BOARD!

Dear reader, dear friend,

Welcome to what could well be the most exciting book you will ever read!

A paradise for the lazy student to instantly improve his memory and grades, and an incredible opportunity for all the readers to find happiness by managing to achieve the goals that really count for them.

We are all gathered around the same topic: concentration.

***

In the first part of this book, you will discover that concentration is by far the most efficient way to reach success. Anyone who succeed carries within himself a great power of concentration.

You will see that concentration depends exclusively on two levers:

- The first lever is your knowledge of the best practices. In other words, <u>the good 'technical rules'</u> that enhance concentration (like good organization, good preparation, good stress management etc.).

- The second lever is <u>your natural ability to concentrate</u>.

***

So, the second part of the book is dedicated to the first lever: the best practices. You will discover the most efficient practices and rules to improve drastically your concentration.

All of these best practices have been developed by the world top Doctors and Experts in personal efficiency, to ensure you the highest quality of information.

Because good information is in general difficult to find, everything you have to know about the best practices lies here:

A treasure made of precious and well guarded gems to acquire a power of concentration that will give you an advantage almost unfair over others, especially if you are a <u>little bit lazy or a really lazy student</u>.

***

The third part of the book is dedicated to the second lever: your natural ability to concentrate. This is by far the most important of the two levers, but this is also the most ignored.

And yet, <u>the real secret of concentration lies here</u>.

Indeed, the world most successful people ALL had an incredible natural ability to concentrate.

But what less than 1% of people know is that this ability is not necessarily innate.

More than that, it can be widely improved by using some jealously kept techniques or disclosed only to a few privileged people.

The Doctor Vittoz secret concentration technique is one of them, and was widely used by one of the most important contributor to humanity: Albert Einstein.

This technique will improve your memory in all fields, and the results you will get may change your life.

Like Einstein himself said when he saw the results: "The Vittoz will revolutionize the World".

***

HOW TO USE THIS BOOK

Here is how to use this book in 2 steps:

1- Read the book in the order in which it was written for best efficiency.

2- Put into practice what you are about to discover.

The respect of these 2 rules is crucial for your success.

***

Now, let's start immediately, and...

... May the power of concentration transform your life for the best!

Part 1- A NEW BEGINNING IN LIFE WITH EINSTEIN'S SECRET

a- *Concentration: the Key to Success*

> *"Wealthy men and women are noted for their power of concentration"*, Don King.

Concentration is the great secret of power and success. Studies have revealed this surprising fact: on a sample of people who succeed in their life (success in the broad sense, that is they reached a goal they set for themselves, whether it is to become rich, to ace a difficult exam or to be successful at a certain skill, etc.), ALL had incredible focus ability. Their particularity was that in any condition, even the most difficult (ambient noise, stressful situations, limited furniture or financial resources etc.), these people remained fully concentrated.

But let's have a closer look on what concentration really means.

The Merriam-Webster defines the action of concentrating as "a directing of the attention or of the mental faculties toward a single object".

So, concentration gives you the power to both:

1- achieve a specific goal in your life

AND

2- fully concentrate on what you want as long as you want.

1- Achieve a specific goal in your life.

You may ask yourself:

"Why so many people are not able to achieve goals that really count for them?".

The reason is because they are not able to remain exclusively focused on their goals enough time.

Indeed, 97% of the people almost always drift from their goal day after day, because they start thinking at early stage about a back-up plan…just in case that something fails!

In other words, they are adopting one of the most common and efficient way to fail: they are unconsciously anticipating failure by "putting their eggs in several baskets".

On the contrary, successful people can demonstrate enough concentration power to dedicate themselves to the attainment of their goal with an unswerving singleness of purpose.

They know how to keep the main thing the main thing, no matter the goal they want to achieve nor the amount of time they set for it (a day, a month, a year…).

As Andrew Carnegie said: "put all your eggs in one basket and watch the basket".

Being able to concentrate exclusively and enough time on the goal you want to achieve is the only way that will lead you to success.

2- Fully concentrate on what you want as long as you want.

This point is about concentration applied to short durations -from several minutes up to several hours-.

That's why this point is generally fascinating for students (High-School, College or University students) because it directly concerns lectures, study time and... success at exams!

Indeed, a good concentration gives a student the power to both reduce his study time by 3 or more AND improve significantly his grades at the same time. (This book will reveal you precisely how to do this).

Here are the reasons of what is claimed here:

***

Why a good concentration can reduce your study time by 3 or more:

First, because a high concentration state will allow you to get rid of distractions during your study time and to stay exclusively focused on the content of your study.

Thus, you will be able to resize your study-time slots and make them shorter, because they will be free from these time-wasting moments of distraction.

Second, because good concentration automatically triggers good memorization. Which means the more concentrated you are during a lecture, the more information you will memorize, and the less study time you will need because you won't have to memorize this information again.

Believe it or not, but anyone who has a 100% locked-in attention during a lecture is able to restitute at least 87% of the lecture in details.

So, there's a lot to bet that very soon, your actual study-time slots will become oversized, as if you were in a shirt really too large for you.

***

Why concentration can improve your grades:

During an exam or an admission test, you need to make the most of every minute because a ¼ of points can make all the difference between you and another student.

That's why having a high concentration level is crucial, because you can't afford losing a single minute dreaming or thinking about something with absolutely no link with your exam.

Moreover, a high concentration increases drastically the speed of your thinking process: you are able to recall an information or to do a calculation at least twice faster than if your mind is constantly interrupted.

Thus, your performance soars and you automatically increase your chances to get better grades and to have an advantage over others in an entrance exam.

b- Examples of Successful People with Incredible Focus Ability

***

Albert Einstein is naturally one of them.

His concentration ability led him to become one of the most fascinating and influential figures of the modern era with his unique contribution to modern physics.

***

Napoleon had naturally an extraordinary high degree of concentration.

He could jump with the greatest ease from one work to another, without being disturbed by his previous work and completely mind-free to start the next one.

His day finished, he could sleep very soundly at night even amidst busy war, and wake up a few hours later with the same immediacy and completely rested.

Napoleon's power of concentration was so enormous that he impressed people with the quality of his memory for detail and facts.

Indeed, it is argued that when on campaign in 1805 one of his subordinates could not locate his division.

While his aids searched through maps and papers, the Emperor informed the officer of his unit's present location, where he would be for the next three nights, the status and resume of the units strength as well as the subordinates military record.

This out of an army with seven corps, a total of 200,000 men, with all the units on the move.

***

Beethoven was twenty years old when he became deaf.

Yet, he wrote only splendid compositions because his deafness gave him the power of total concentration and the ability to hear his music in his own mind.

***

At the capture of Syracuse by the Romans, **Archimede** was drawing up on the ground a defense plan to protect the city.

He was so concentrated on his drawing that, even with the chaos that reigned in the city and the cries of distress of his fellow-citizens, he didn't notice the averse army forces a few steps behind him.

He was killed by an enemy without even seeing him.

c- The Lazy Student's Golden Concentration Formula

As specified previously, concentration can be defined by the following formula:

***

$$\text{CONCENTRATION} = BP \times (NAC)^2$$

Where:

BP stands for **'Best Practices'**
NAC stands for **'Natural Ability to Concentrate'**

***

This means that your concentration directly depends on the 'Best Practices' (BP) to apply and your Natural Ability to Concentrate (NAC).

So, just let the Best Practices of this book guide you and the Doctor Vittoz secret technique activate your untapped concentration ability, and watch a miracle happen in your life!

Part 2- EXPERTS BEST PRACTICES TO IMPROVE THE LAZY STUDENT'S CONCENTRATION

<u>Best Practice 1</u>: HOW TO INSTANTLY RECOVER YOUR POWER OF CONCENTRATION WHEN YOU FEEL STRESSED OR ANXIOUS

Stress, worries and anxiety can directly impact your ability to concentrate, and thus your ability to memorize things.

When your are under stress conditions, you may feel your mind foggy and sometimes sloppy, as if you were in another place, not really present.

In such conditions, it is essential to regain a clear mind before being able to concentrate again.

Here is a very particular breathing technique developed by the world renowned expert in personal efficiency Philippe Morando, with **particularly beneficial effects**.

Your anxiety, fears, negative thoughts will disappear instantly each time you will use this breathing.

You can use this special breathing any time of the day, whenever you feel stressed and need to relax or to confront situations that require having a complete self-control.

In a couple of minutes, your inner peace and calm will be restored as efficiently as a deep meditation.

This technique has the advantage to be simple and discreet.

So, you can use it anywhere, at any moment without anybody noticing.

You can be in a standing or sitting position, or lying down on the back.

If you chose a sitting position, your arms and your legs should not be crossed. Take care that your body can loosen without falling or moving.

***

PROCEDURE FOR THE SPECIAL BREATHING

Initial condition: Mouth should be closed during all the phases.

1- First phase: Breathing in.

Length: in general 4 seconds minimum.

First take a deep breath through the nose, without forcing. Hearing the sound of the air in your nostrils proves the breath you took is correct: vigorous but without roughness.

While your lungs are filling with air, the air will naturally push forward your diaphragm and also your belly. It is important here not to force to push forward your belly. Let things happen naturally. Your belly will be pushed forward by itself.

After several times, you could try to take a little more air than the first times. When you reach your maximum, still try to take a little bit more air: trying to increase the capacity of your ribcage will have a massaging action on the solar plexus and thus it will relax your nerves.

2- Second phase: Intermediate phase.

Length: about 3 seconds.

When your lungs are completely filled with air, try to keep the air for about 3 seconds, then you can loosen everything. Don't force yourself to keep the air too long: 3 seconds are enough in general.

3- Third phase: Breathing out.

Length: in general about 6 seconds.

Your lungs empty themselves. You breathe out through the nose. Don't force to remove the air from your lungs. The air will get out of your lungs naturally.

The breathing out should be like a relaxation, **a loosening**. Don't try to empty completely your lungs. The air should get out naturally without your help like a balloon that deflates. No matter if it remains a little bit air in your lungs.

<u>Note:</u> *This phase of breathing out is a loosening phase. So, each time you breathe out, you can add a small sound of relief like "hummm" (mouth still closed). By this sound, you show your determination to let yourself go.*

4- Fourth phase: Resting phase.

Length: From 2 to 10 seconds and even more.

At the end of the breathing out, you may not feel the need to start to breathe again immediately. So, keep this state with lungs almost empty, without looking for breathing again right now. Enjoy this state of **well-being**.

When you **want to breathe in** again, and only at this moment, start again the phase 1.

***

You can do 2 or 3 special breathings whenever you need.

You can also do 5 minutes of this special breathing in the morning when you wake up, and 5 minutes in the evening before falling asleep.

You will then create a very good habit in the long term: your breathing will become better during the day, and you could notice that you will adopt spontaneously this special breathing during the difficult moments of the day.

SUMMARY OF THE 4 PHASES OF THE SPECIAL BREATHING

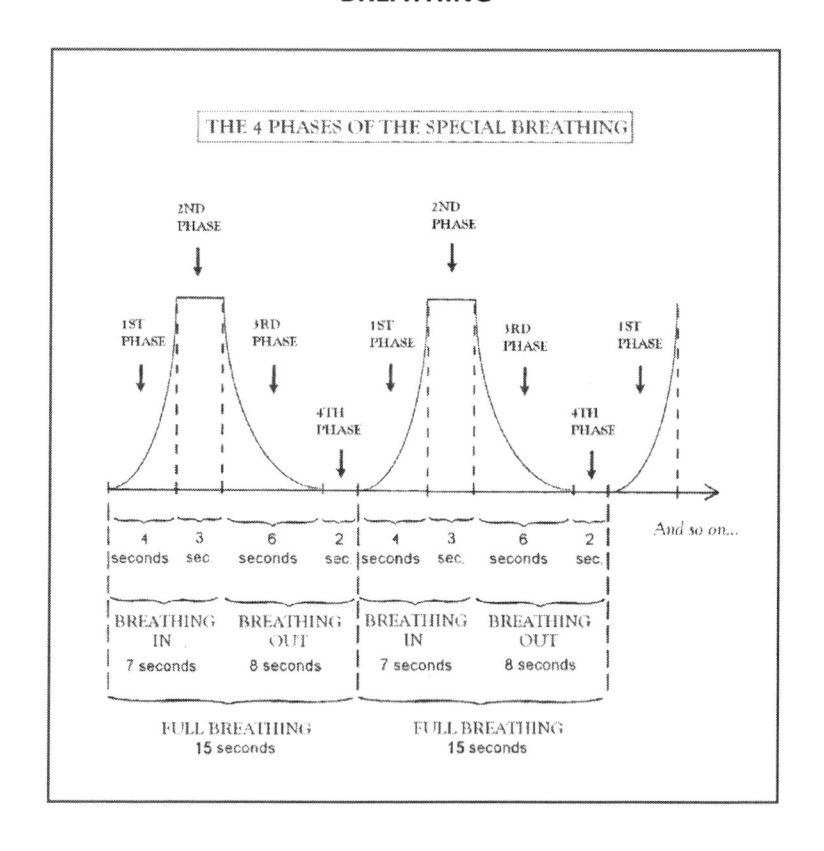

THE 4 PHASES OF THE SPECIAL BREATHING

1ST PHASE	2ND PHASE	3RD PHASE	4TH PHASE
4 seconds	3 sec.	6 seconds	2 sec.

- BREATHING IN — 7 seconds
- BREATHING OUT — 8 seconds

FULL BREATHING — 15 seconds

And so on...

Best Practice 2: HOW TO CONCENTRATE TO REDUCE YOUR STUDY TIME BY 3 OR MORE AND INSTANTLY INCREASE YOUR EFFICIENCY

If you are a student, you surely know one or two students who give an incredible impression of being always relaxed, always free for a baseball game or a party. They never seem to be working so much and yet, they almost always get good grades!

This is partly due to the fact that they know how to manage their study time efficiently when they study alone and don't depend on a teacher or a lecturer.

This allows them to have a maximum concentration during a minimum amount of time.

Thus, they have more free time and get much better results compared to other students who work for hours late in the evening.

Here are the best students' secrets to manage your study time when you study alone:

SECRET 1- SET A PRECISE HOUR FOR YOUR STUDY AND RESPECT IT

It is essential that you create one very good habit: to study at the same time every day.

It will accustom your brain to be focused and concentrated on your study at a given moment.

How can you find your own moment for your study?

Just have a look at the timetable of one of your typical week. Then, choose the hour where you are free every day.

There is not a strict rule concerning a potential 'best hour' to study. The best hour will be simply the one you prefer!

It can be early in the morning or in the evening. Just make sure you have enough time to sleep, for example if you decide to study between 5h30 to 7h00 a.m.

Indeed, sleeping plays an important role in the memorization process. It is during your sleep that your brain organizes and stores all the information you learned during the day.

Before you continue, note here the moment you chose to study every day.

**"Every day, I will study from:
…….h……. to …….h……."**

Now, the only thing you have to do is to respect what you wrote just above.

Respect the moment you chose and don't change this moment every week.

You will know that you are on the road to your success when you will be able to stop your favorite TV show just because it is the time you set for your study: This is one of the winners' secrets.

You will then appreciate the new comfort of life this organization brings you, and you could enjoy how free is your mind during the rest of the day!

SECRET 2-HOW TO MAKE THE MOST OF YOUR STUDY PERIODS

Once you set precisely your study periods with the tool just above, you will now want to be as efficient as possible during this moment.

To do this, it is psychologically essential to spend a few minutes to determine **what you want** and **how much time you have to acquire it**.

You can find this by answering these 2 questions:

a-What knowledge do you want to acquire by this work?

AND

b-How much time do you have in order to do this work?

a-What knowledge do you want to acquire by this work?

Here, you are setting a goal in order to focus your brain and memory to find the information you want.

With a goal, the brain and the memory work much better because they exactly know what must be found and memorized.

This step is very important, don't neglect it.

So, answer this question as precisely as possible, and **write down your answer**.

For instance, if you want to study Ernest HEMINGWAY, don't just write a general answer like: "I want to know Ernest HEMINGWAY", but prepare a list of what you want to know about him, even if you want to know everything.

b-How much time do you have in order to do this work?

Before answering this second question, you have to know that:

**The more time we HAVE,
the more time we TAKE.**

Often unnecessarily.

This principle has been verified thousands of times and illustrates perfectly that **the brain acts in the limits it is given**.

It can be also known as the Parkinson's law: "Work expands so as to fill the time available for its completion."

It means that if you give yourself 2 hours to do a work, it is likely that you will spend 2 hours. If you give yourself 3 hours for the same work, you will surely spend 3 hours.

Your work will be often better with less time because it will appear easier (except if the time allocated is really too short). Indeed, the more the amount of time spent on a work is large, the more this work will appear as being voluminous and complex.

Moreover, **taking less time will force you to get rid of distractions**.

It will put you under a high concentration state in order to remain focused on the essential.

So, instead of asking yourself how much time you have to do a work, it is much better to ask yourself in how much time **YOU decide** to do this work.

EVEN IF IT SEEM SURPRISING, REMEMBER THAT IS IS POSSIBLE TO WORK BOTH QUICKLY AND WELL.

<u>On condition that you follow a clear and precise plan, and that you know exactly what you want to obtain and in how much time.</u>

SET YOURSELF goals and you will make great strides in your life.

SECRET 3-TAKE REGULAR BREAKS

Tiredness is a cause of inattention and can happen to everyone, even to people who have a good attention in general.

If you feel tired, it is likely that you won't be able to concentrate correctly and there is no need to insist too much.

You should really avoid working to the point of exhaustion and you should take regular breaks while you are studying.

A break that lasts 4 or 5 minutes is enough.

The general rule is that one hour and half of intellectual work should be a maximum to not overpass without taking a break.

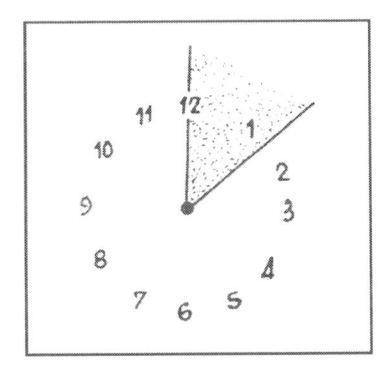

BUT THE BEST IS TO TAKE A SHORT BREAK EVERY 45 MINUTES.

Best Practice 3: HOW YOUR STUDY PLACE CAN INCREASE YOUR CONCENTRATION BY 27% AND MORE IN TWO SIMPLE STEPS

STEP 1:
HOW TO CREATE A COMFORTABLE AND WELCOMING STUDY PLACE

Your study place should be comfortable and welcoming enough to make you feel good when you are there.

***

Comfort starts by **choosing a good chair**. If the chair is not comfortable, it will induce pain and interfere with your studying.

If the chair is too comfortable, it will make you sleepy and also interfere with your studying.

Select a chair on which you can sit and maintain your attention for long periods.

***

To make your study place more welcoming and cheerful (without being eccentric), you can **play with colors**.

However be careful, there are some notions to know concerning the symbolism of colors:

RED

Symbol of fire, blood and conquest. It strongly stimulates the nervous system.

ORANGE

Linked to emotions. It is less stimulating than red and gives a more welcoming and cozy atmosphere.

YELLOW

Refers to light, evokes material and spiritual wealth. Yellow symbolizes the energy of a bright sunny day. It awakes and mobilizes the body and mind but without being over-stimulating like red.

GREEN

Depending on its dominant proportion of yellow or blue, it can be either a warm or cold color. It is the most restful color for the nervous system and it symbolizes peace. That is why you can find a lot of green in games like billiard or in conference rooms. The nature also provides more green than stimulating colors.

BLUE

It is a cold and calming color. It is associated with night, sleep and relaxation.

INDIGO & PURPLE

With a predominance of blue, purple is the symbol of the union between the man and the sacred. A predominance of red symbolizes the power of the earthly reign (purple of kings, judicial robe).

***

You also have to take into account the temperature of colors.

Cold colors like green, blue and purple are calming.

Warm colors like red, orange and yellow stimulate more the eyes and can be seen from farther away.

For instance, it will be hard for you to concentrate on a book put on a red surface. Your eyes will be permanently attracted by this red color and your nervous system will be more and more excited.

It is very important that you have only cold or neutral colors in your field of vision while studying: blue, green, white, beige, very pale yellow (mat and not glossy), brown.

Naturally, you can use all the range of these colors, from the lightest to the darkest.

***

STEP 2:
HOW TO KEEP YOUR DESK TIDY

Being tidy will make you save your energy as well as your time.

The German poet Goethe wrote:

"Order will teach you how to win time."

Work with care and you will win time. You will avoid a lot of mistakes by being tidy.

Working roughly will make you lose time, because you will have to start your work again, to come back to the previous chapter, to search something for a second time.

Follow this famous rule widely used in business management strategy: "A place for everything, and everything in its place."

Give to each object of your working material a determined place. Don't think it is a kind of fussiness, it is just efficiency.

For example, imagine you are studying and you are very concentrated on what you are learning. Your attention is at its highest level.

Suppose that at a precise moment, you need to take a ruler and a pencil to draw a line.

If you know exactly their place, you just hold out your hand, take them and continue your work. You keep your concentration intact and unchanged.

Imagine now the same scenario: you hold out your hand to take the ruler and...no ruler!

So, you have to stop your work and try to remember where could be the famous ruler...

After several wasted minutes, you start to become angry and above all, you have lost for good your concentration state.

That is why you have to know the exact place of each object of your working material.

When you need something, you should be able to have it instantly so that you keep your concentration at its highest level.

When you do not need the object any more, put it at the same place you took it.

You can for example place together objects of the same nature to remember more easily their location.

Best Practice 4: *HOW TO AVOID GETTING DISTRACTED BY PEOPLE, TV AND OTHER SPARE-TIME ACTIVITIES AND REMAIN FOCUSED*

The moment when you study should be exclusively yours.

This moment belongs to you, to the success of your exam and you will want to be exclusively focused on your study without permitting anything and anyone to distract you.

That is why refuse to be disturbed.

If possible, the best is to be alone during the time of your study. So, during this moment, everyone has to consider that you are not at home and not available.

Tell people who live with you that during X time you are not here and that they have to act as if you were missing.

Switch off your mobile phone, deactivate online chats, social networks and anything that could disturb you during your study.

Television and radio should be naturally also switched off. It is wrong to think that a background noise can help to concentrate. It is only a habit some people took and they are no longer aware of it. It can only reduce their ability to concentrate.

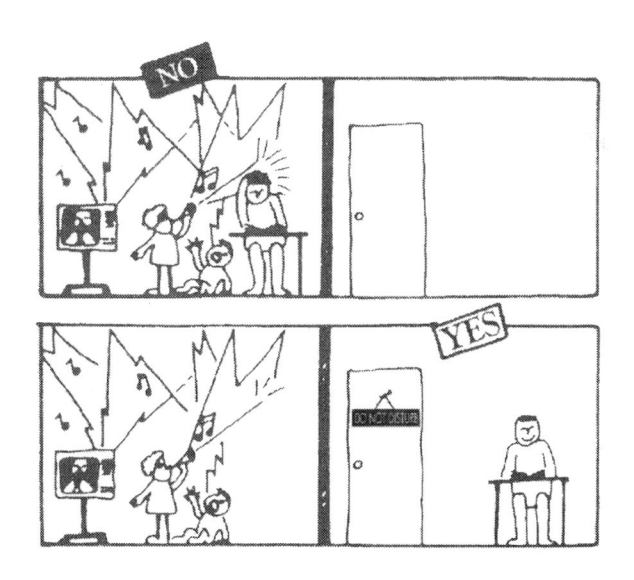

Best Practice 5: *HOW TO INSTANTLY STOP YOUR MIND FROM WANDERING WHEN YOU NEED TO CONCENTRATE*

During a lecture or while you are studying, your mind may drift off and you may start thinking about something totally different (for example a movie, an upcoming event, your lunch etc...).

If you tend being distracted like this, it is essential to solve this problem as soon as possible.

Indeed, a lot people complain about their bad memory.

In reality, the problem is not their memory but their lack of attention.

If you have difficulties to memorize, this often means that you haven't paid enough attention at what you read, heard or studied.

For instance, imagine yourself starting a bus city tour in a city you have never been before.

During the tour, your cell phone rings and you start a deep conversation in order to organize the birthday party of your best friend.

You are totally absorbed by the conversation and you don't pay attention to any detail during the tour.

Result: When the tour ends, you are practically unable to remember what you saw: the different monuments, places, streets names, shops, squares...

Your attention was not focused on the tour: your mind was somewhere else.

So, for not getting distracted and instantly stop your mind from wandering, follow this golden rule:

ELIMINATE IMMEDIATELY ANY INTRUSIVE THOUGHT

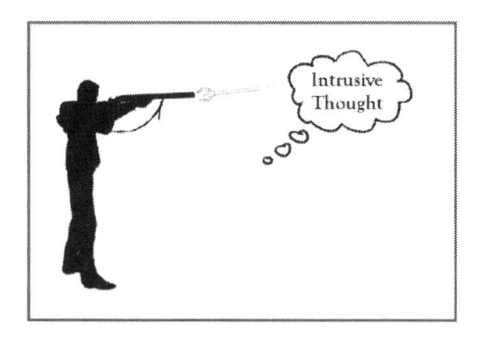

As soon as a thought with no link with your study comes to your mind, eliminate it immediately.

Even if this thought is pleasant.

To manage to eliminate it, <u>return immediately</u> on the topic of your study.

<u>This will create an excellent habit.</u>

Little by little, you will see that the frequency of intrusive thoughts will be close to zero, even if they were very frequent at the beginning.

Best Practice 6: *HOW TO KEEP A FULL CONCENTRATION DURING A THREE HOURS LECTURE*

Here is how to proceed:

BEFORE THE LECTURE

A few seconds before the beginning of a lecture, you should prepare yourself to have a 100% locked-in concentration. Here is how to proceed, just let the 5 simple steps below guide you:

A) Naturally, you will want to avoid talking unnecessarily during the lecture. So, try to avoid sitting next to talkative people, in particular some talkative friends.

B) Mentally, take stock of your knowledge on the subject of the lecture. This will allow you to find one or several comparison points that will help you to memorize new information.

C) Relax and do a few deep breathings (using the special breathing technique described in the Best Practice 1 is perfect here). Try to sit comfortably.

D) Just before the beginning, as soon as the lecturer appears, close your eyes. Cut yourself off from your environment and concentrate.

E) As soon as the lecturer starts to talk, open your eyes and keep your eyes focused on him, only on him, until the end.

ACT AS IF YOU WERE ALONE WITH THE LECTURER AND THE NOTHINGNESS ALL AROUND.

DURING THE LECTURE

The secret is to have an **attitude as active as possible** during a lecture. If the teacher asks a question, try to answer it. It will increase your interest and thus your attention.

LOOK instead of just seeing.

During the lecture, pay a particular attention to every drawing, graphic or scheme that the teacher can make.

Pictures are memorized better than words and are excellent 'hooks' for the memory: they are perfect aids for memorizing easily any concept that refers to them.

So, every time you see a picture, a scheme or graphic, pay attention to it. Copy it and write down some brief explanations next to it.

Have a general look on each picture, scheme or graphic. What kind of concept or situation does it refers to? Then, have a closer look on its details.

LISTEN instead of just hearing.

At the same time, listen carefully to the explanations of the teacher. So, take only brief notes to avoid getting distracted too long and to keep your attention focused on the teacher's explanations.

If you don't understand something, try to understand it as soon as possible. Indeed, you can't focus your attention for a long time on something you don't understand.

So, try to have an explanation from your teacher immediately.

If it is difficult (if there are too many students), write a fast note or a symbol (for example the symbol '?') next to the point you don't understand and ask your teacher an explanation at the end of the lecture.

Part 3- THE DOCTOR VITTOZ SECRET CONCENTRATION TECHNIQUE

Here we are!

You are about to be revealed the secret concentration technique developed by the Swiss Doctor Vittoz, widely used by Einstein himself.

This technique will develop your Natural Ability to Concentrate (NAC), and has been specially developed for people who are unable to concentrate.

It will progressively train your mind to concentrate, and will widely contribute to improve your memory in all fields.

If you practice it seriously and regularly, you should start to see some great improvements within a few days.

In a couple of weeks (in general 17 days or less), your natural ability to concentrate should have improved so greatly that you will surprise your friends, your family, your teachers and...yourself!

Indeed, this technique gives you the power to concentrate on what you want as long as you want.

So, let's start **RIGHT NOW**!

THE DOCTOR VITTOZ SECRET CONCENTRATION TECHNIQUE

The technique consists in several series of small exercises to practice frequently if you have problems of attention.

The exercises are very quick to do.

If possible, do them several times a day. You will soon notice with pleasure that your attention has improved drastically.

Warning:

DO NOT START THE NEXT SERIES OF EXERCISES BEFORE YOU COMPLETELY MASTER THE PREVIOUS ONE

If needed, you can practice a series longer than another one.

1rst SERIES

Exercise n°1

Eyes closed, imagine a row of trees on each side of a road. Follow with your eyes these 2 rows, starting from the trees closest to you up to the farthest (when the 2 rows seem to merge into a single point at infinity).

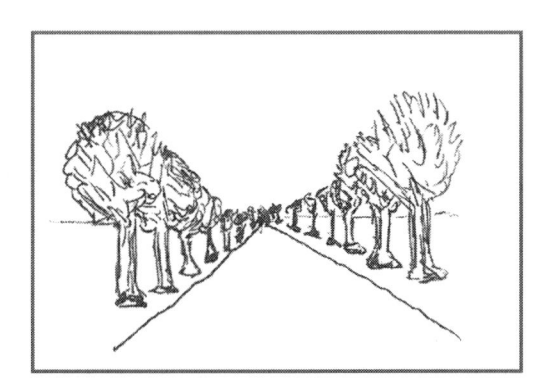

Exercise n°2

Eyes closed, imagine a child on a swing. Follow the movement of the swing slowing down, until it totally stops.

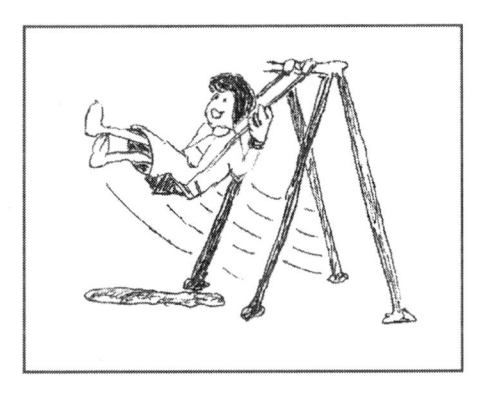

Exercise n°3

Eyes closed, imagine a train stopped. On the last wagon is drawn the letter i on a large white panel.

Follow the movement of this letter i when the train starts, and watch this letter becoming smaller and smaller until it becomes only a point.

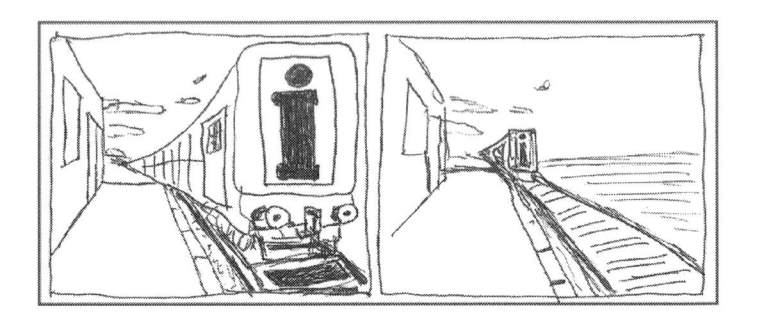

2nd SERIES

Exercise n°1

Eyes open, draw in the air the sign of infinity with your right forefinger.

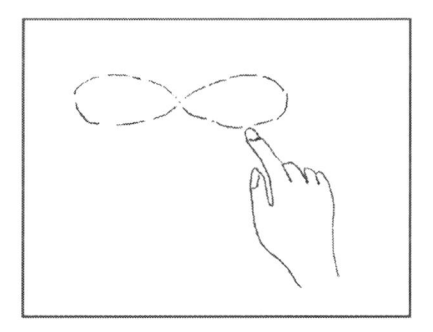

Then, draw the same sign with your left forefinger.

Repeat theses 2 movements with eyes closed.

Then, keep the eyes closed and draw mentally this sign without moving your hands.

Exercise n°2

Eyes open, draw in the air 2 spirals simultaneously with your 2 forefingers:

First, both spirals from left to right.

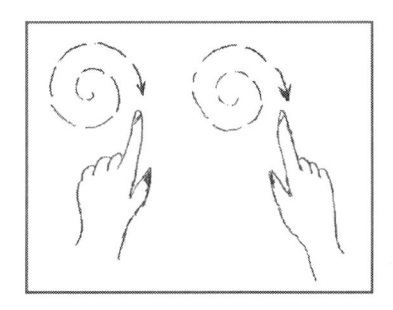

Then, both spirals from right to left.

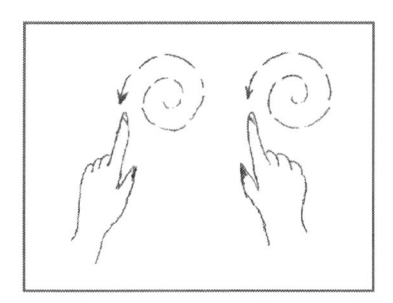

56

Then, each spiral in a different direction.

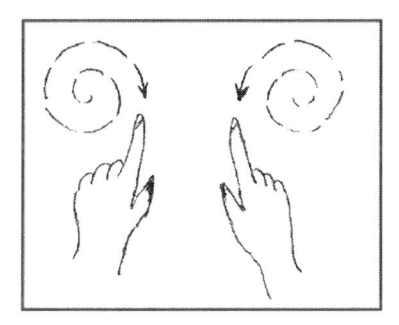

Finally, each spiral in the opposite direction.

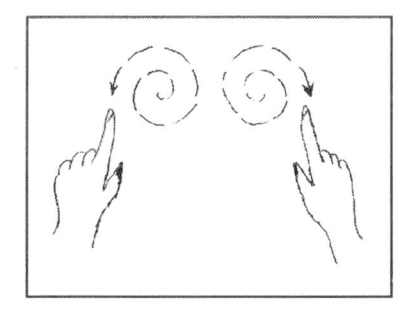

Repeat these exercises the eyes closed.

Then, repeat them again mentally without using your hands.

Exercise n°3

Eyes closed, imagine a flower in bud. You see the flower opening and blossoming in a slow and steady movement.

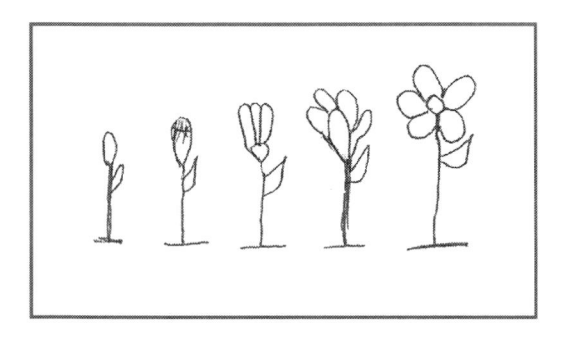

Simultaneously, relax and feel you fulfill yourself like the flower.

3rd SERIES

Exercise n°1

Put eight to ten different objects on a table. Remove them one by one, starting from the last one you put.

Repeat this exercise mentally: eyes closed, imagine the objects on the table and eliminate them one by one.

Exercise n°2

Eyes closed, imagine you are writing on a blackboard the number 1, then the number 2 and finally the number 3.

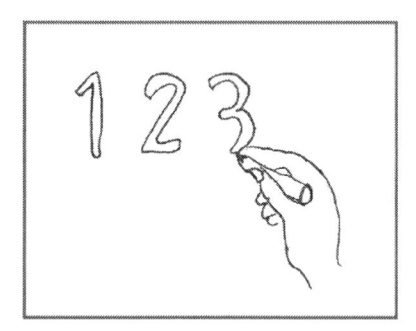

When you visualize them well, erase them starting from the 3, then the 2 and finally the 1.

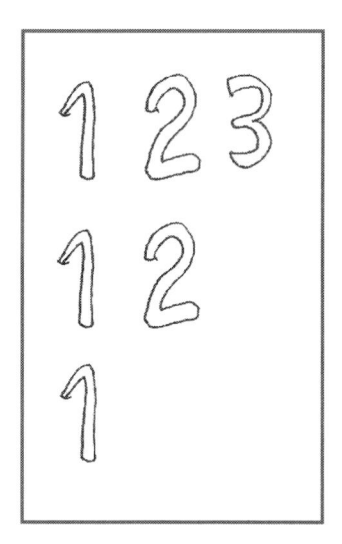

60

Exercise n°3

Eyes closed, imagine you are writing on a blackboard the word NEW YORK.

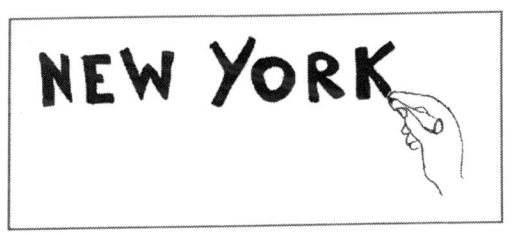

NEW YORK

Once you visualize it well, erase the K, the R, the O, the Y, the W, the E and the N.

NEW YORK
NEW YOR
NEW YO
NEW Y
NEW
NE
N

61

4th SERIES

Exercise n°1

Relax and close your eyes. Start ten deep breathings and concentrate on the path the air takes in your throat and lungs while you breathe in and out.

Exercise n°2

Relax, close your eyes and breathe slowly. Count 1 at the 1st breath in, 2 at the 1st breath out, 3 at the 2nd breath in, 4 at the 2nd breath out etc...until 20.

Exercise n°3

Relax and close your eyes. Breathe slowly ten times, and try not to think about something else.

ONE LAST WORD

Dear reader, dear friend,

You have now finished this book. Above all, remember to put into practice what you learned.

I hope you enjoyed it, and that it will bring you the success and the happiness in life you really deserve.

**I WISH YOU ALL THE BEST FROM
THE BOTTOM OF MY HEART.**

REMY ROULIER

ABOUT THE AUTHOR

Remy Roulier is a former computer science engineer and marketing manager in a multinational company. He is now a digital nomad and travels around the world, and has gained over the last ten years a strong expertise in Internet marketing and self development.

He now shares his tools and experience to help others achieve their financial independence and design their life as they truly and deeply want it to be.

MORE BOOKS FROM THE AUTHOR

RESCUE ACUPRESSURE:
INSTANTLY SUPPRESS STRESS, HEADACHES, MEMORY LAPSES IN DESPERATE SITUATIONS LIKE DURING AN EXAM
Relieve pain and discomfort immediately when you need it and do not let them make you fail an exam, a job interview or any important moment of your life. 100% practical, very clear and simple, this book is definitely the best investment you can do for your health and success.

DETOX DIET:
EATING WELL FOR A LIFE OF PURE ENERGY, SHAPE AND HEALTH
All you need to know about eating well to get an exceptional health and shape is inside this book. Discover now the true principles to eating well (4 powers and 4 poisons) that will completely detoxify you and allow you to create an exceptional health, shape, and energy.

You can also find dozens of other books in French from the author on Amazon.

Printed in Poland
by Amazon Fulfillment
Poland Sp. z o.o., Wrocław